A Beginner Guide to Your Diabetic diet Meals

Many recipes to prepare as a family

for a special lunch or a sweet dessert

Roseann Smith

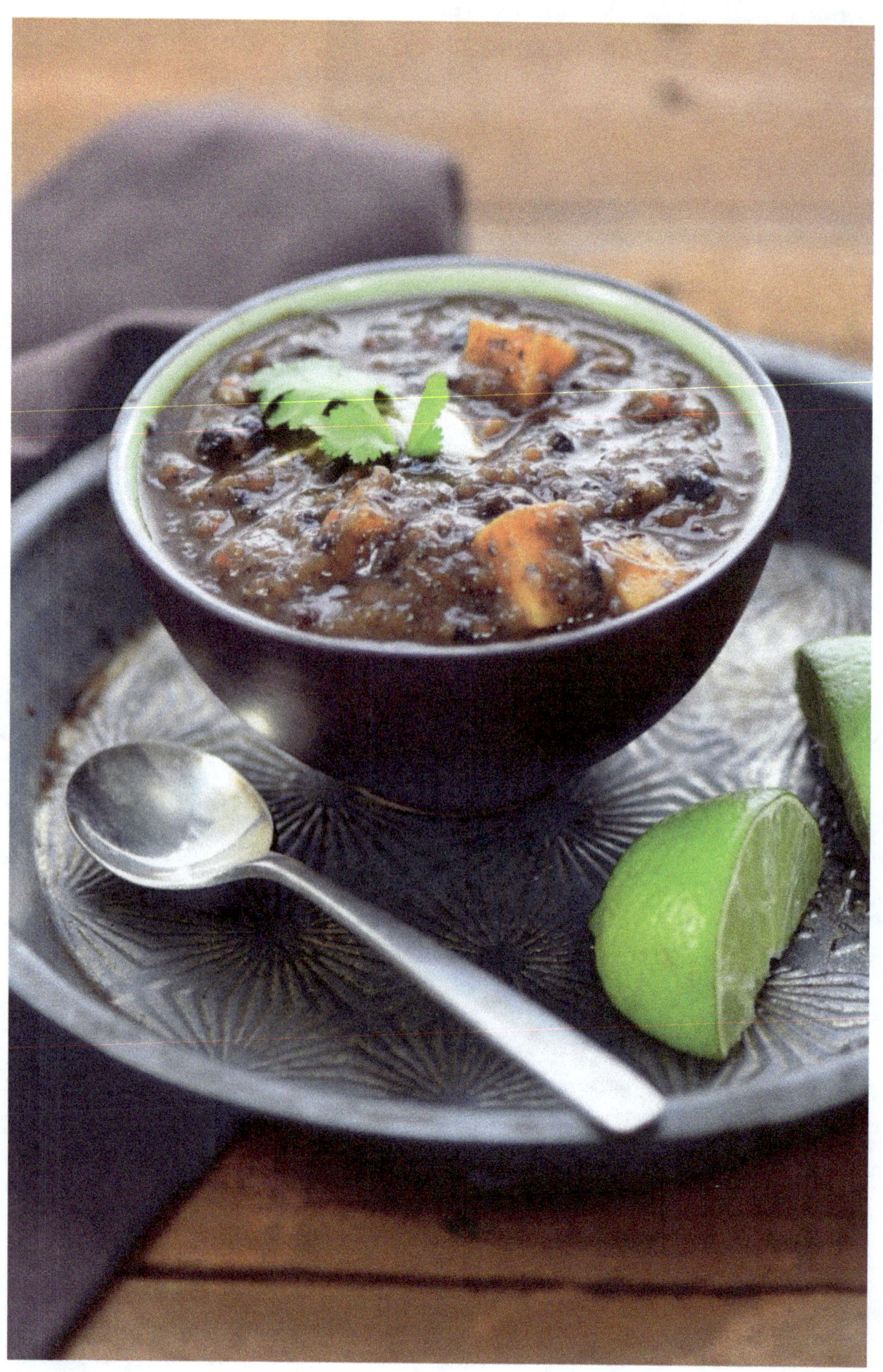

Disclaimer Notice:

Please note the information contained within this document is for educational and entertainment purposes only. All effort has been executed to present accurate, up to date, and reliable, complete information. No warranties of any kind are declared or implied. Readers acknowledge that the author is not engaging in the rendering of legal, financial, medical or professional advice. The content within this book has been derived from various sources. Please consult a licensed professional before attempting any techniques outlined in this book.

By reading this document, the reader agrees that under no circumstances is the author responsible for any losses, direct or indirect, which are incurred as a result of the use of information contained within this document, including, but not limited to, — errors, omissions, or inaccuracies.

Table of Contents

Easy Beef Stew 6

Chicken Bacon Soup 8

Rhubarb Stew 11

Buffalo Chicken Soup 13

Chinese Tofu Soup... 15

Healthy Spinach Soup 17

Cream Of Tomato Soup 19

Tasty Basil Tomato Soup 20

Fake-on Stew.. 22

Coconut Chicken Soup 23

Herb Tomato Soup.. 27

Flavorful Broccoli Soup 29

Beef And Cabbage Soup 31

Shiitake Soup 33

Sausage & Turnip Soup 35

Simple Chicken Soup 37

Black Bean Soup 40

Thick Creamy Broccoli Cheese Soup 42

Delicious Chicken Soup 44

Chicken And Dill Soup 46

Broccoli Stilton Soup 48

Creamy Broccoli Cauliflower Soup 50

Zoodle Won-ton Soup 52

Pumpkin Spice Soup 54

Kidney Bean Stew 56

Cream Zucchini Soup..57

Spinach & Basil Chicken Soup 60

Easy Wonton Soup 62

Lemon Fat Bombs 64

Garden Patch Sandwiches On Multigrain Bread................66

Sesame Almond Fat Bombs 68

Sugar Free Carrot Cake 70

Spice Cake...73

Creamy Chocolate Pie Ice Pops 76

Caramel Popcorn..78

Tiramisu Shots 80

Fruit Kebab 82

Cheese Berry Fat Bomb 84

Tamari Toasted Almonds...85

Choco Peppermint Cake 87

Frozen Lemon & Blueberry 89

Pumpkin & Banana Ice Cream..91

Coconut Chia Pudding...93

Strawberries In Honey Yogurt Dip 95

Mortadella & Bacon Balls 97

Lemon Cake... 100

Green Fruity Smoothie.. 103

Baked Creamy Custard With Maple 105

Lemon Cookies 107

Pineapple Nice Cream 110

Easy Beef Stew

Servings: 6

Cooking Time: 5 Minutes

Ingredients:

- 1 shredded green cabbage head
- 4 chopped carrots
- 2 ½ lbs. non-fat beef brisket
- 3 chopped garlic cloves
- Black pepper
- 2 bay leaves
- 4 c. low-sodium beef stock

Directions:

1. Put the beef brisket in a pot, add stock, pepper, garlic and bay leaves, provide your simmer over medium heat and cook for an hour.

2. Add carrots and cabbage, stir, cook for a half-hour more, divide into bowls and serve for lunch.

3. Enjoy!

Nutrition Info: Calories: 271, Fat:8 g,Carbs:16 g, Protein:9 g, Sugars:3.4 g, Sodium:760 mg

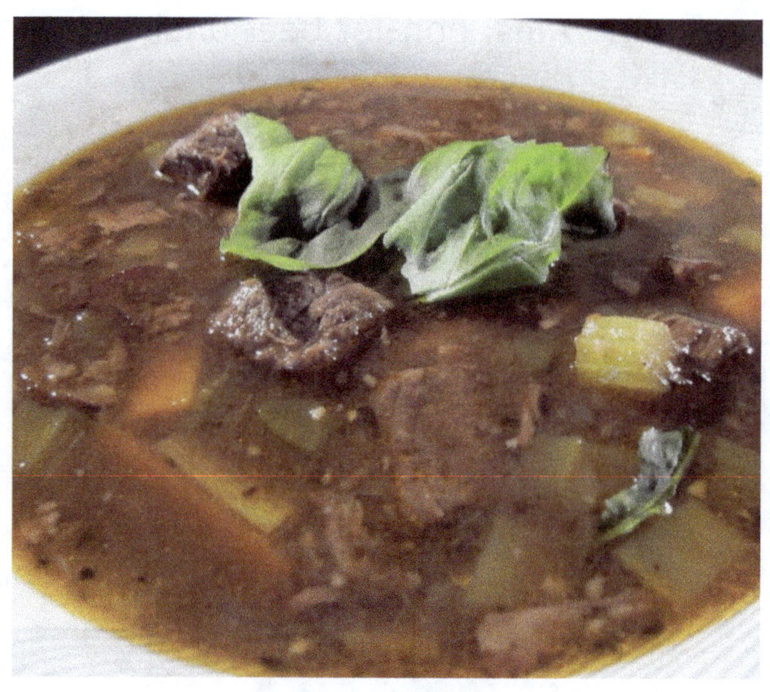

Chicken Bacon Soup

Servings: 4

Cooking Time: 40 Minutes

Ingredients:

- 6 boneless, skinless chicken thighs, make cubes
- ½ cup chopped celery
- 4 minced garlic cloves
- 6-ounce mushrooms, sliced
- ½ cup chopped onion
- 8-ounce softened cream cheese
- ¼ cup softened butter
- 1 teaspoon dried thyme
- Salt and (finely ground) black pepper, as per taste preference
- 2 cups chopped spinach
- 8 ounces cooked bacon slices, chopped

- 3 cups (preferably homemade) chicken broth
- 1 cup heavy cream

Directions:

1. Arrange Instant Pot over a dry platform in your kitchen. Open its top lid and switch it on.

2. Add the ingredients except for the cream, spinach, and bacon; gently stir to mix well.

3. Close the lid to create a locked chamber; make sure that safety valve is in locking position.

4. Find and press "SOUP" cooking function; timer to 30 minutes with default "HIGH" pressure mode.

5. Allow the pressure to build to cook the ingredients.

6. After cooking time is over press "CANCEL" setting. Find and press "NPR" cooking function. This setting is for the

natural release of inside pressure and it takes around 10 minutes to slowly release pressure.

7. Slowly open the lid, stir in cream and spinach.

8. Take out the cooked in serving plates or serving bowls and enjoy the keto. Top with the bacon.

Nutrition Info: Calories - 456 Fat: 38g Saturated Fat: 13g Trans Fat: 0g Carbohydrates: 7g Fiber: 1g Sodium: 742mg Protein: 23g

Rhubarb Stew

Servings: 3

Cooking Time: 10 Minutes

Ingredients:

- 1 tsp. grated lemon zest
- 1 ½ c. coconut sugar
- Juice of 1 lemon
- 1 ½ c. water
- 4 ½ c. roughly chopped rhubarbs

Directions:

1. In a pan, combine the rhubarb while using water, fresh lemon juice, lemon zest and coconut sugar, toss, bring using a simmer over medium heat, cook for 5 minutes, and divide into bowls and serve cold.

2. Enjoy!

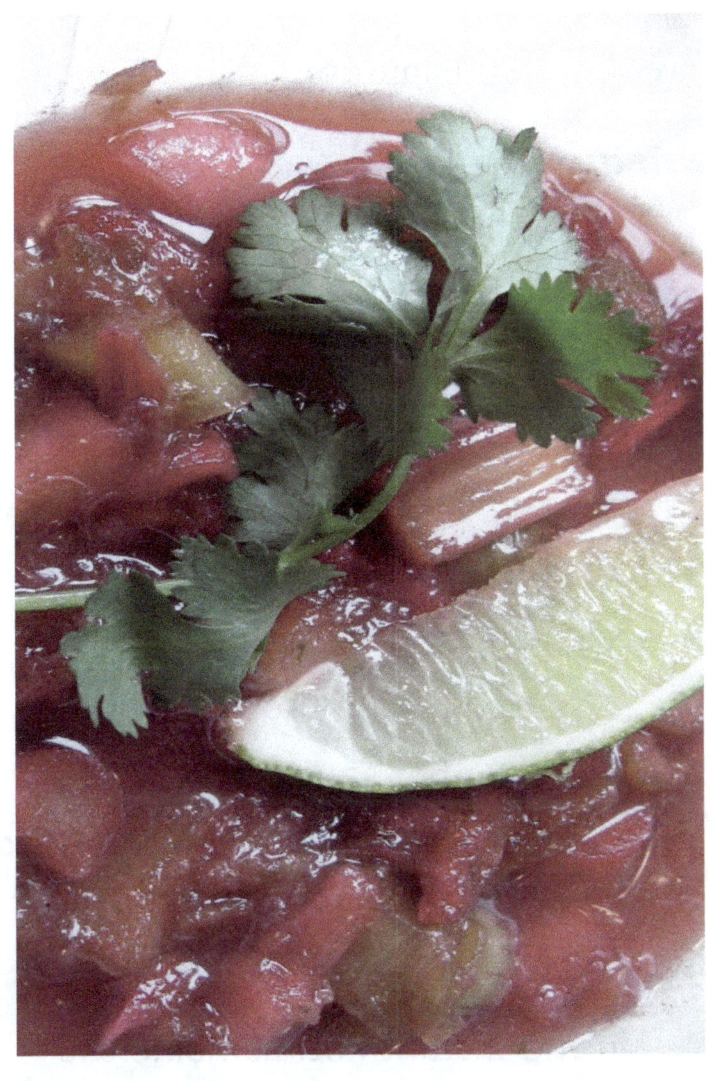

Buffalo Chicken Soup

Servings: 8

Cooking Time: 30 Minutes

Ingredients:

- 2 chicken breasts, boneless, skinless, frozen or fresh
- 1 clove garlic, chopped
- ¼ cup onion, diced
- ½ cup celery, diced
- 2 tbsp butter
- 1 tbsp ranch dressing mix
- 3 cups chicken broth
- 1/3 cup hot sauce
- 2 cups cheddar cheese, shredded
- 1 cup heavy cream

Directions:

1. In the Instant Pot, combine the chicken breasts, garlic, onion, celery,

butter, ranch dressing mix, broth, and hot sauce.

2. Close and lock the lid. Select MANUAL and cook at HIGH pressure for 10 minutes.

3. Once cooking is complete, let the pressure Release Naturally for 10 minutes. Release any remaining steam manually. Uncover the pot.

4. Transfer the chicken to a plate and shred the meat. Return to the pot.

5. Add the cheese and heavy cream. Stir well. Let sit for 5 minutes and serve.

Nutrition Info: Calories 303 Fat 27.5 g Carbohydrates 13.8 g Sugar 5 g Protein 4.g Cholesterol 33 mg

Chinese Tofu Soup

Servings: 2

Cooking Time: 10 Minutes

Ingredients:

- 2 cups chicken stock
- 1 tbsp soy sauce, sugar-free
- 2 spring onions, sliced
- 1 tsp sesame oil, softened
- 2 eggs, beaten
- 1-inch piece ginger, grated
- Salt and black ground, to taste
- ½ pound extra-firm tofu, cubed
- A handful of fresh cilantro, chopped

Directions:

1. Boil in a pan over medium heat, soy sauce, chicken stock and sesame oil. Place in eggs as you whisk to incorporate completely. Change heat to

low and add salt, spring onions, black pepper and ginger; cook for 5 minutes. Place in tofu and simmer for 1 to 2 minutes.

2. Divide into soup bowls and serve sprinkled with fresh cilantro.

Nutrition Info: Calories 163; Fat: 10g, Net Carbs: 2.4g, Protein: 14.5g

Healthy Spinach Soup

Servings: 8

Cooking Time: 3 Hours

Ingredients:

- 3 cups frozen spinach, chopped, thawed and drained
- 8 oz cheddar cheese, shredded
- 1 egg, lightly beaten
- 10 oz can cream of chicken soup
- 8 oz cream cheese, softened

Directions:

1. Add spinach to a large bowl. Purée the spinach.
2. Add egg, chicken soup, cream cheese, and pepper to the spinach purée and mix well.
3. Transfer spinach mixture to a crock pot.

4. Cover and cook on low for 3 hours.

5. Stir in cheddar cheese and serve.

Nutrition Info: Calories 256 Fat 21.9 g Carbohydrates 4.1 g Sugar 0.5 g Protein 11.1 g Cholesterol 84 mg

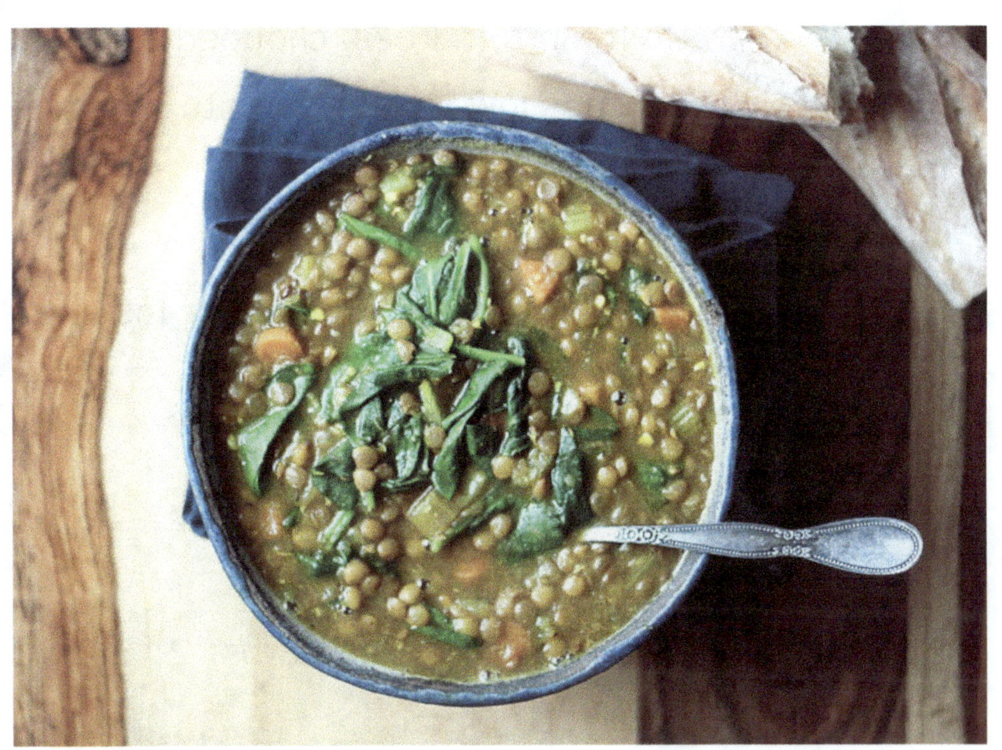

Cream Of Tomato Soup

Servings: 2

Cooking Time: 15 Minutes

Ingredients:

- 1lb fresh tomatoes, chopped
- 1.5 cups low sodium tomato puree
- 1tbsp black pepper

Directions:

1. Mix all the ingredients in your Instant Pot.
2. Cook on Stew for 15 minutes.
3. Release the pressure naturally.
4. Blend.

Nutrition Info: Calories: 20; Carbs: 2; Sugar: 1; Fat: 0; Protein: 3; GL: 1

Tasty Basil Tomato Soup

Servings: 6

Cooking Time: 6 Hours

Ingredients:

- 28 oz can whole peeled tomatoes
- 1/2 cup fresh basil leaves
- 4 cups chicken stock
- 1 tsp red pepper flakes
- 3 garlic cloves, peeled
- 2 onions, diced
- 3 carrots, peeled and diced
- 3 Tbsp olive oil
- 1 tsp salt

Directions:

1. Add all ingredients to a crock pot and stir well.
2. Cover and cook on low for 6 hours.

3. Purée the soup until smooth using an immersion blender.

4. Season soup with pepper and salt.

5. Serve and enjoy.

Nutrition Info: Calories 126 Fat 7.5 g Carbohydrates 13.3 g Sugar 7 g Protein 2.5 g Cholesterol 0 mg

Fake-on Stew

Servings: 2

Cooking Time: 25 Minutes

Ingredients:

- 0.5lb soy bacon
- 1lb chopped vegetables
- 1 cup low sodium vegetable broth
- 1tbsp nutritional yeast

Directions:

1. Mix all the ingredients in your Instant Pot.
2. Cook on Stew for 25 minutes.
3. Release the pressure naturally.

Nutrition Info: Calories: 200; Carbs: 12; Sugar: 3; Fat: 7; Protein: 41; GL: 5

Coconut Chicken Soup

Servings: 4

Cooking Time: 18 Minutes

Ingredients:

- 4 cloves of garlic, minced
- 1-pound chicken breasts, skin-on
- 4 cups of water
- 2 tablespoons olive oil
- 1 onion, diced
- 1 cup of coconut milk
- (finely ground) black pepper and salt as per taste preference
- 2 tablespoons sesame oil

Directions:

1. Arrange Instant Pot over a dry platform in your kitchen. Open its top lid and switch it on.

2. Find and press "SAUTE" cooking
    function; add the oil in it and allow it to
    heat.

3. In the pot, add the onions, garlic; cook
    (while stirring) until turns translucent
    and softened for around 1-2 minutes.

4. Stir in the chicken breasts; stir, and
    cook for 2 more minutes.

5. Pour in water and coconut milk —
    season to taste.

6. Close the lid to create a locked
    chamber; make sure that safety valve
    is in locking position.

7. Find and press "MANUAL" cooking
    function; timer to 15 minutes with
    default "HIGH" pressure mode.

8. Allow the pressure to build to cook the
    ingredients.

9. After cooking time is over press
    "CANCEL" setting. Find and press "NPR"
    cooking function. This setting is for the

natural release of inside pressure and it takes around 10 minutes to slowly release pressure.

10. Slowly open the lid, Drizzle with sesame oil on top.

11. Take out the cooked in serving plates or serving bowls and enjoy the keto.

Nutrition Info: Calories - 328 Fat: 31g Saturated Fat: 6g Trans Fat: 0g Carbohydrates: 6g Fiber: 4g Sodium: 76mg Protein: 21g

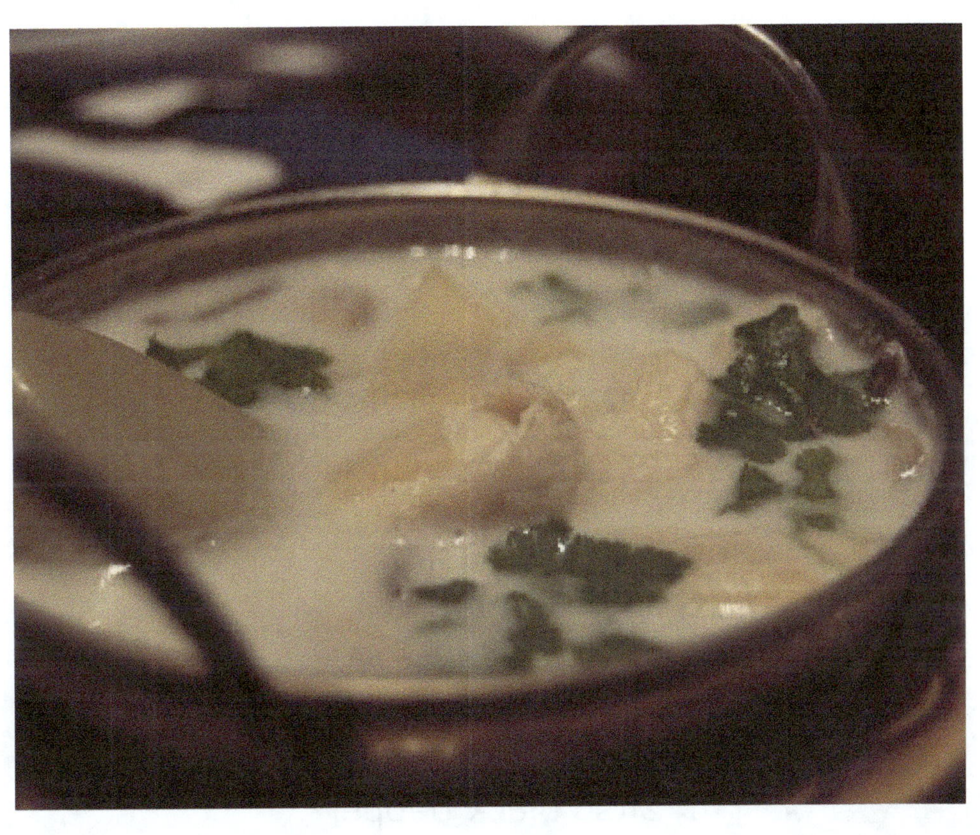

Herb Tomato Soup

Servings: 8

Cooking Time: 6 Hours

Ingredients:

- 55 oz can tomatoes, diced
- 1/2 onion, minced
- 2 cups chicken stock
- 1 cup half and half
- 4 Tbsp butter
- 1 bay leaf
- 1/2 tsp black pepper
- 1/2 tsp garlic powder
- 1 tsp oregano
- 1 tsp dried thyme
- 1 cup carrots, diced
- 1/4 tsp black pepper
- 1/2 tsp salt

Directions:

1. Add all ingredients to a crock pot and stir well.
2. Cover and cook on low for 6 hours.
3. Discard bay leaf and purée the soup using an immersion blender until smooth.
4. Serve and enjoy.

Nutrition Info: Calories 145 Fat 9.4 g Carbohydrates 13.9 g Sugar 7.9 g Protein 3.2 g Cholesterol 26 mg

Flavorful Broccoli Soup

Servings: 6

Cooking Time: 4 Hours 15 Minutes

Ingredients:

- 20 oz broccoli florets
- 4 oz cream cheese
- 8 oz cheddar cheese, shredded
- 1/2 tsp paprika
- 1/2 tsp ground mustard
- 3 cups chicken stock
- 2 garlic cloves, chopped
- 1 onion, diced
- 1 cup carrots, shredded
- 1/4 tsp baking soda
- 1/4 tsp salt

Directions:

1. Add all ingredients except cream cheese and cheddar cheese to a crock pot and stir well.
2. Cover and cook on low for 4 hours.
3. Purée the soup using an immersion blender until smooth.
4. Stir in the cream cheese and cheddar cheese.
5. Cover and cook on low for 15 minutes longer.
6. Season with pepper and salt.
7. Serve and enjoy.

Nutrition Info: Calories 275 Fat 19.9 g Carbohydrates 11.9 g Sugar 4 g Protein 14.4 g Cholesterol 60 mg

Beef And Cabbage Soup

Servings: 6

Cooking Time: 35 Minutes

Ingredients:

- 2 tbsp coconut oil
- 1 onion, diced
- 1 clove garlic, minced
- 1 lb ground beef
- 14 oz can diced tomatoes, undrained
- 4 cups water
- Salt and ground black pepper to taste
- 1 head cabbage, chopped

Directions:

1. Preheat the Instant Pot by selecting SAUTÉ. Add and heat the oil.
2. Add the onion and garlic and sauté for 2 minutes.

3. Add the beef and cook, stirring, for 2-3
    minutes until lightly brown.
4. Pour in the water and tomatoes.
    Season with salt and pepper, stir well.
5. Press the CANCEL key to stop the
    SAUTÉ function.
6. Close and lock the lid. Select MANUAL
    and cook at HIGH pressure for 12
    minutes.
7. When the timer goes off, use a Quick
    Release. Carefully open the lid.
8. Add the cabbage, select SAUTÉ and
    simmer for 5 minutes.
9. Serve.

Nutrition Info: Calories 335 Fat 10 g
Carbohydrates 13.6 g Sugar 6 g Protein 4.9 g
Cholesterol 33 mg

Shiitake Soup

Servings: 2

Cooking Time: 35 Minutes

Ingredients:

- 1 cup shiitake mushrooms
- 1 cup diced vegetables
- 1 cup low sodium vegetable broth
- 2tbsp 5 spice seasoning

Directions:

1. Mix all the ingredients in your Instant Pot.

2. Cook on Stew for 35 minutes.

3. Release the pressure naturally.

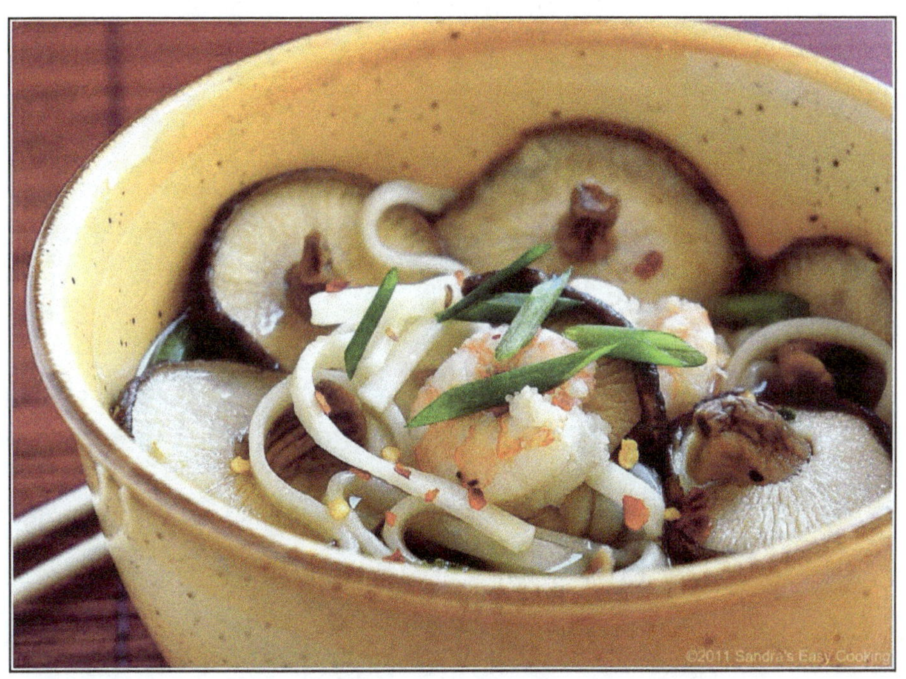

Sausage & Turnip Soup

Servings: 4

Cooking Time: 20 Minutes

Ingredients:

- 3 turnips, chopped
- 2 celery sticks, chopped
- 2 tbsp butter
- 1 tbsp olive oil
- 1 pork sausage, sliced
- 2 cups vegetable broth
- ½ cup sour cream
- 3 green onions, chopped
- 2 cups water
- Salt and black pepper, to taste

Directions:

1. Sauté the green onions in melted butter over medium heat until soft and golden, about 3-4 minutes. Add celery

and turnip, and cook for another 5 minutes. Pour over the vegetable broth and water over.

2. Bring to a boil, simmer covered, and cook for about 20 minutes until the vegetables are tender. Remove from heat. Puree the soup with a hand blender until smooth. Add sour cream and adjust the seasoning. Warm the olive oil in a skillet. Add the pork sausage and cook for 5 minutes. Serve the soup in deep bowls topped with pork sausage.

Nutrition Info: Calories 275, Fat: 23.1g, Net Carbs: 6.4g, Protein: 7.4g

Simple Chicken Soup

Servings: 4

Cooking Time: 25 Minutes

Ingredients:

- 2 frozen, boneless chicken breasts
- 4 medium-sized potatoes, cut into chunks
- 3 carrots, peeled and cut into chunks
- ½ big onion, diced
- 2 cups chicken stock
- 2 cups water
- Salt and ground black pepper to taste

Directions:

1. In the Instant Pot, combine the chicken breasts, potatoes, carrots,

onion, stock, water, salt and pepper to taste.

2. Close and lock the lid. Select MANUAL and cook at HIGH pressure for 25 minutes.

3. Once timer goes off, allow to Naturally Release for 10 minutes, and then release any remaining pressure manually. Uncover the pot.

4. Serve.

Nutrition Info: Calories 301 Fat 27.2 g Carbohydrates 13.6 g Sugar 6 g Protein 4.9 g Cholesterol 33 mg

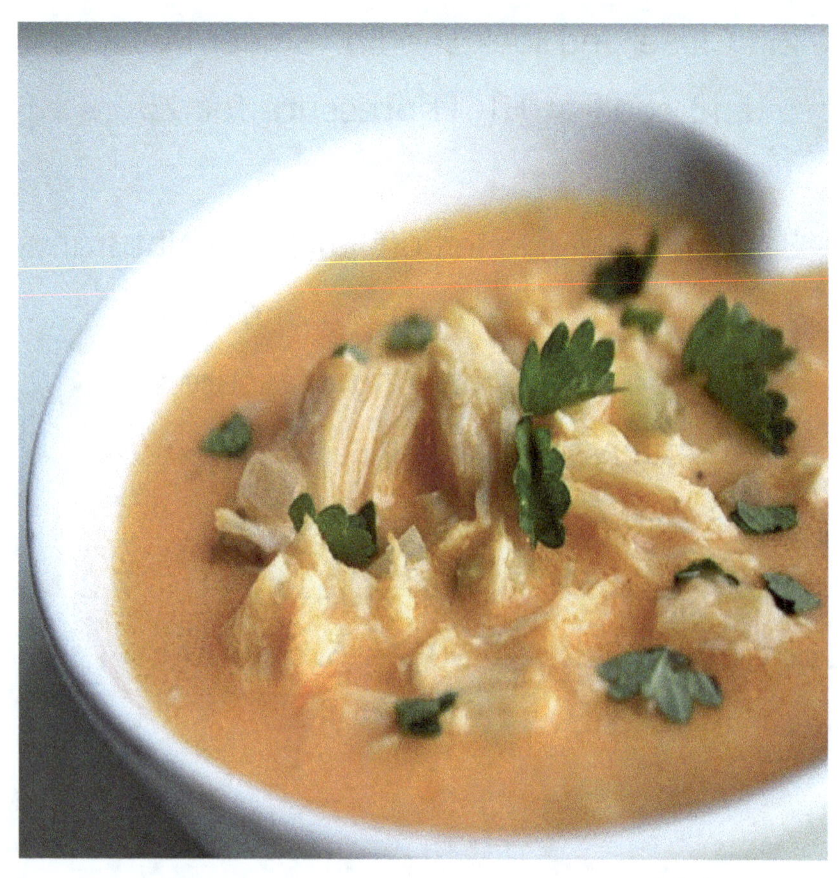

Black Bean Soup

Servings: 4

Cooking Time: 10 Minutes

Ingredients:

- 1 tsp. cinnamon powder
- 32 oz. low-sodium chicken stock
- 1 chopped yellow onion
- 1 chopped sweet potato
- 38 oz. no-salt-added, drained and rinsed canned black beans
- 2 tsps. organic olive oil

Directions:

1. Heat up a pot using the oil over medium heat, add onion and cinnamon, stir and cook for 6 minutes.
2. Add black beans, stock and sweet potato, stir, cook for 14 minutes, puree

utilizing an immersion blender, divide into bowls and serve for lunch.

3. Enjoy!

Nutrition Info: Calories: 221, Fat:3 g,Carbs:15 g, Protein:7 g, Sugars:4 g, Sodium:511 mg

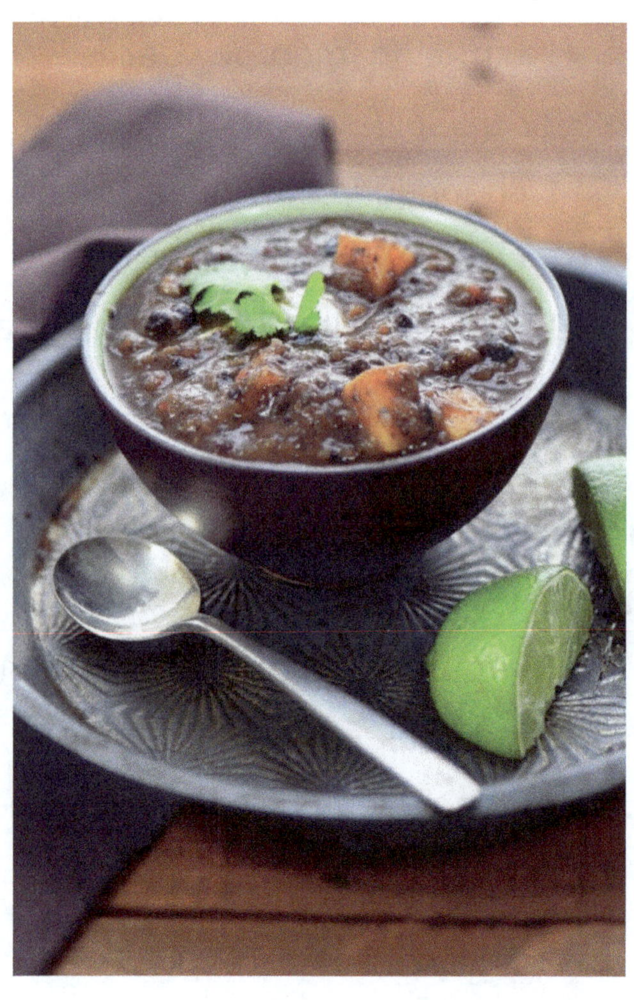

Thick Creamy Broccoli Cheese Soup

Servings: 4

Cooking Time: 10 Minutes

Ingredients:

- 1 tbsp olive oil
- 2 tbsp peanut butter
- ¾ cup heavy cream
- 1 onion, diced
- 1 garlic, minced
- 4 cups chopped broccoli
- 4 cups veggie broth
- 2 ¾ cups cheddar cheese, grated
- ¼ cup cheddar cheese to garnish
- Salt and black pepper, to taste
- ½ bunch fresh mint, chopped

Directions:

1. Warm olive oil and peanut butter in a pot over medium heat. Sauté onion and garlic for 3 minutes or until tender, stirring occasionally. Season with salt and black pepper. Add the broth and broccoli and bring to a boil.

2. Reduce the heat and simmer for 10 minutes. Puree the soup with a hand blender until smooth. Add in the cheese and cook about 1 minute. Stir in the heavy cream. Serve in bowls with the reserved grated cheddar cheese and sprinkled with fresh mint.

Nutrition Info: Calories 552, Fat: 49.5g, Net Carbs: 6.9g, Protein: 25g

Delicious Chicken Soup

Servings: 4

Cooking Time: 4 Hours 30 Minutes

Ingredients:

- 1 lb chicken breasts, boneless and skinless
- 2 Tbsp fresh basil, chopped
- 1 1/2 cups mozzarella cheese, shredded
- 2 garlic cloves, minced
- 1 Tbsp Parmesan cheese, grated
- 2 Tbsp dried basil
- 2 cups chicken stock
- 28 oz tomatoes, diced
- 1/4 tsp pepper
- 1/2 tsp salt

Directions:

1. Add chicken, Parmesan cheese, dried basil, tomatoes, garlic, pepper, and salt to a crock pot and stir well to combine.
2. Cover and cook on low for 4 hours.
3. Add fresh basil and mozzarella cheese and stir well.
4. Cover again and cook for 30 more minutes or until cheese is melted.
5. Remove chicken from the crock pot and shred using forks.
6. Return shredded chicken to the crock pot and stir to mix.
7. Serve and enjoy.

Nutrition Info: Calories 299 Fat 11.6 g Carbohydrates 9.3 g Sugar 5.6 g Protein 38.8 g Cholesterol 108 mg

Chicken And Dill Soup

Servings: 6

Cooking Time: 10 Minutes

Ingredients:

- 1 c. chopped yellow onion
- 1 whole chicken
- 1 lb. sliced carrots
- 6 c. low-sodium veggie stock
- ¼ tsp. black pepper and salt
- ½ c. chopped red onion
- 2 tsps. chopped dill

Directions:

1. Put chicken in a pot, add water to pay for, give your boil over medium heat, cook first hour, transfer to a cutting board, discard bones, shred the meat, strain the soup, get it back on the pot,

heat it over medium heat and add the chicken.

2. Also add the carrots, yellow onion, red onion, a pinch of salt, black pepper and also the dill, cook for fifteen minutes, ladle into bowls and serve.

3. Enjoy!

Nutrition Info: Calories: 202, Fat:6 g, Carbs:8 g, Protein:12 g, Sugars:6 g, Sodium:514 mg

Broccoli Stilton Soup

Servings: 2

Cooking Time: 35 Minutes

Ingredients:

- 1lb chopped broccoli

- 0.5lb chopped vegetables

- 1 cup low sodium vegetable broth

- 1 cup Stilton

Directions:

1. Mix all the ingredients in your Instant Pot.

2. Cook on Stew for 35 minutes.

3. Release the pressure naturally.

4. Blend the soup.

Nutrition Info: Calories: 280; Carbs: 9;

Sugar: 2; Fat: 22; Protein: 13; GL: 4

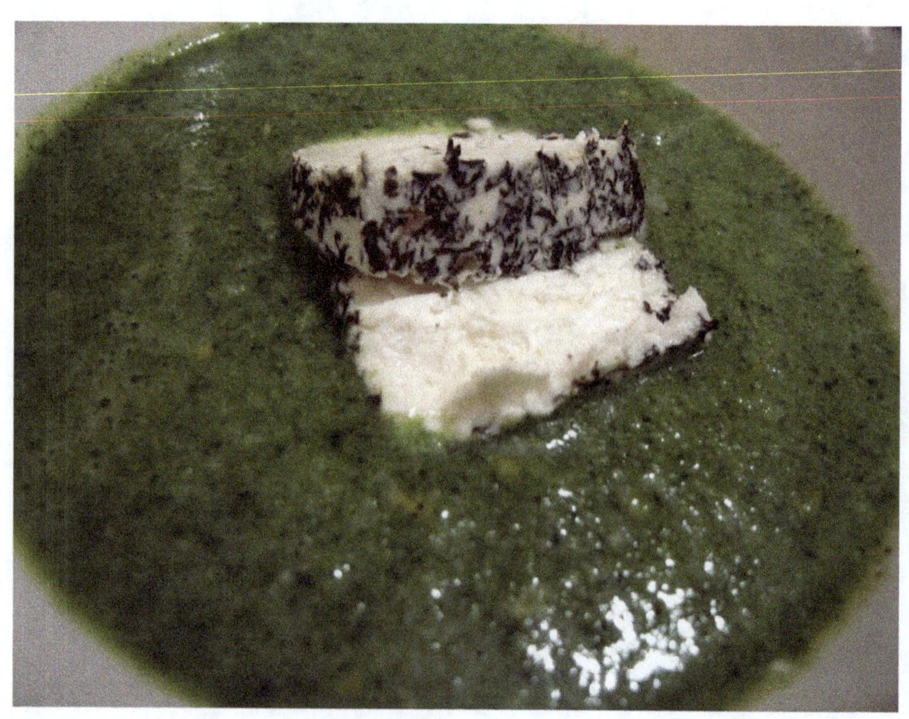

Creamy Broccoli Cauliflower Soup

Servings: 6

Cooking Time: 6 Hours

Ingredients:

- 2 cups cauliflower florets, chopped
- 3 cups broccoli florets, chopped
- 3 1/2 cups chicken stock
- 1 large carrot, diced
- 1/2 cup shallots, diced
- 2 garlic cloves, minced
- 1 cup plain yogurt
- 6 oz cheddar cheese, shredded
- 1 cup coconut milk
- Pepper
- Salt

Directions:

1. Add all ingredients except milk, cheese, and yogurt to a crock pot and stir well.
2. Cover and cook on low for 6 hours.
3. Purée the soup using an immersion blender until smooth.
4. Add cheese, milk, and yogurt and blend until smooth and creamy.
5. Season with pepper and salt.
6. Serve and enjoy.

Nutrition Info: Calories 281 Fat 20 g Carbohydrates 14.4 g Sugar 6.9 g Protein 13.1 g Cholesterol 32 mg

Zoodle Won-ton Soup

Servings: 2

Cooking Time: 5 Minutes

Ingredients:

- 1lb spiralized zucchini

- 1 pack unfried won-tons

- 1 cup low sodium beef broth

- 2tbsp soy sauce

Directions:

1. Mix all the ingredients in your Instant Pot.

2. Cook on Stew for 5 minutes.

3. Release the pressure naturally.

Nutrition Info: Calories: 300; Carbs: 6; Sugar: 1; Fat: 9; Protein: 43; GL: 2

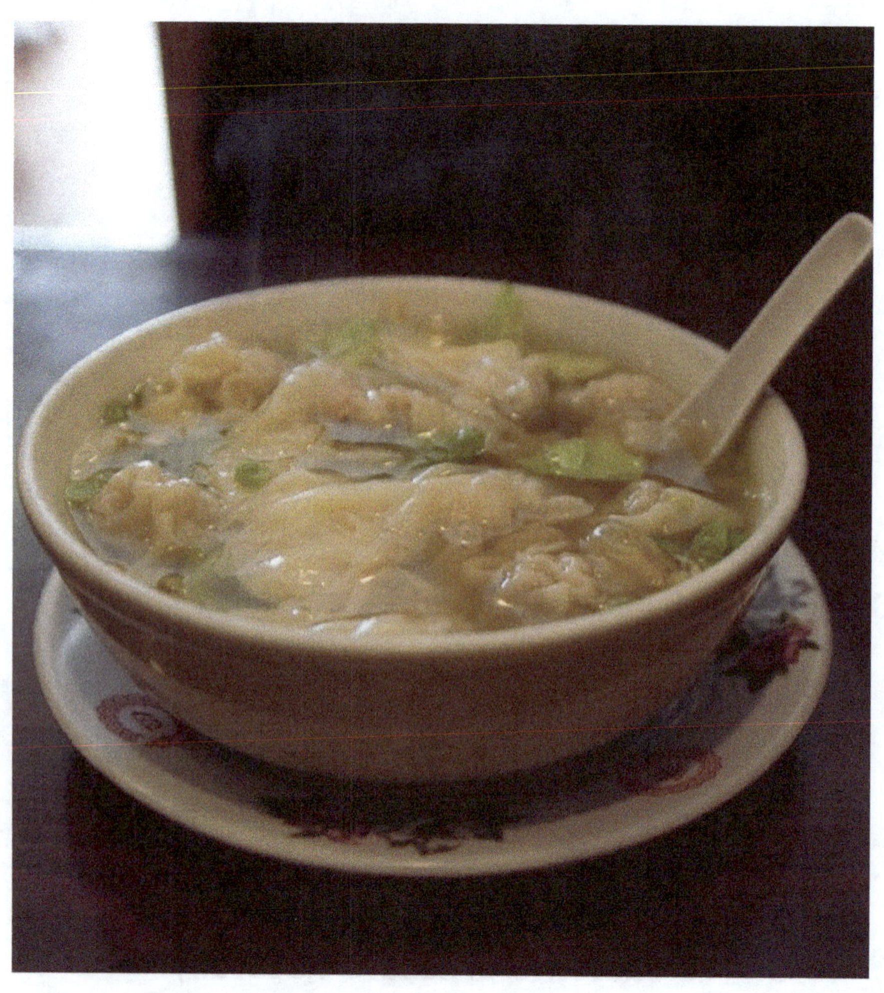

Pumpkin Spice Soup

Servings: 2

Cooking Time: 35 Minutes

Ingredients:

- 1lb cubed pumpkin

- 1 cup low sodium vegetable broth

- 2tbsp mixed spice

Directions:

1. Mix all the ingredients in your Instant

    Pot.

2. Cook on Stew for 35 minutes.

3. Release the pressure naturally.

4. Blend the soup.

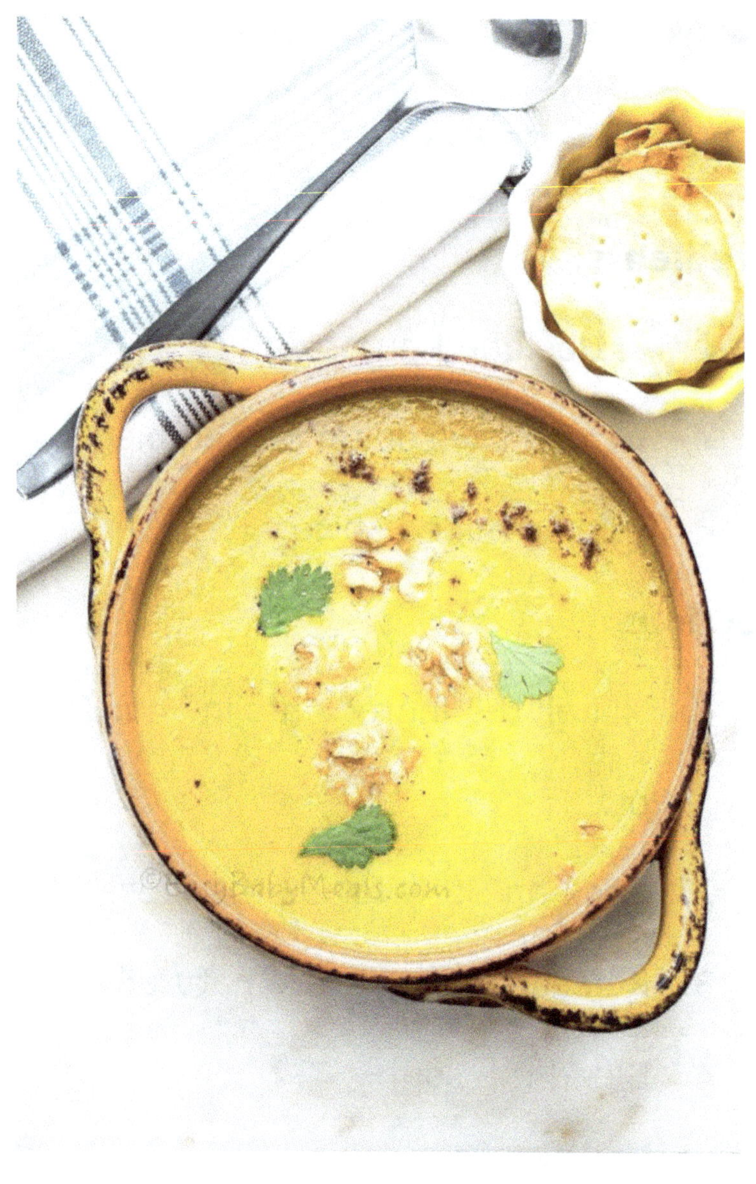

Kidney Bean Stew

Servings: 2

Cooking Time: 15 Minutes

Ingredients:

- 1lb cooked kidney beans
- 1 cup tomato passata
- 1 cup low sodium beef broth
- 3tbsp Italian herbs

Directions:

1. Mix all the ingredients in your Instant Pot.
2. Cook on Stew for 15 minutes.
3. Release the pressure naturally.

Nutrition Info: Calories: 270; Carbs: 16; Sugar: 3; Fat: 10; Protein: 23; GL: 8

Cream Zucchini Soup

Servings: 4

Cooking Time: 8 Minutes

Ingredients:

- 2 cups vegetable stock
- 2 garlic cloves, crushed
- 1 tablespoon butter
- 4 (preferably medium size) zucchinis, peeled and chopped
- 1 small onion, chopped
- 2 cups heavy cream
- 1/2 teaspoon dried oregano, (finely ground)
- 1/2 teaspoon black pepper, (finely ground)
- 1 teaspoon dried parsley, (finely ground)
- 1 teaspoon of sea salt

- Lemon juice (optional)

Directions:

1. Arrange Instant Pot over a dry platform in your kitchen. Open its top lid and switch it on.

2. Find and press "SAUTE" cooking function; add the butter in it and allow it to melt.

3. In the pot, add the onions, zucchini, garlic; cook (while stirring) until turns translucent and softened for around 2-3 minutes.

4. Add the vegetable broth and sprinkle with salt, oregano, pepper, and parsley; gently stir to mix well.

5. Close the lid to create a locked chamber; make sure that safety valve is in locking position.

6. Find and press "MANUAL" cooking function; timer to 5 minutes with default "HIGH" pressure mode.

7. Allow the pressure to build to cook the ingredients.

8. After cooking time is over press "CANCEL" setting. Find and press "QPR" cooking function. This setting is for quick release of inside pressure.

9. Slowly open the lid, take out the cooked in serving plates or serving bowls, and enjoy the keto . Top with some lemon juice.

Nutrition Info: Calories - 264 Fat: 26g Saturated Fat: 7g Trans Fat: 0g Carbohydrates: 11g Fiber: 3g Sodium: 564mg Protein: 4g

Spinach & Basil Chicken Soup

Servings: 4

Cooking Time: 10 Minutes

Ingredients:

- 1 cup spinach
- 2 cups cooked and shredded chicken
- 4 cups chicken broth
- 1 cup cheddar cheese, shredded
- 4 ounces' cream cheese
- ½ tsp chili powder
- ½ tsp ground cumin
- ½ tsp fresh parsley, chopped
- Salt and black pepper, to taste

Directions:

1. In a pot, add the chicken broth and spinach, bring to a boil and cook for 5-8 minutes. Transfer to a food processor, add in the cream cheese and pulse until

smooth. Return the mixture to a pot and place over medium heat. Cook until hot, but do not bring to a boil.

2. Add chicken, chili powder, and cumin and cook for about 3-5 minutes, or until it is heated through.

3. Stir in cheddar cheese and season with salt and pepper. Serve hot in bowls sprinkled with parsley.

Nutrition Info: Calories 351, Fat: 22.4g, Net Carbs: 4.3g, Protein: 21.6g

Easy Wonton Soup

Servings: 6

Cooking Time: 20 Minutes

Ingredients:

- 4 sliced scallions
- ¼ tsp. ground white pepper
- 2 c. sliced fresh mushrooms
- 4 minced garlic cloves
- 6 oz. dry whole-grain yolk-free egg noodles
- ½ lb. lean ground pork
- 1 tbsp. minced fresh ginger
- 8 c. low-sodium chicken broth

Directions:

1. Place a stockpot over medium heat. Add the ground pork, ginger, and garlic and sauté for 5 minutes. Drain any excess fat, then return to stovetop.

2.   Add the broth and bring to a boil. Once boiling, stir in the mushrooms, noodles, and white pepper. Cover and simmer for 10 minutes.

3.   Remove pot from heat. Stir in the scallions and serve immediately.

Nutrition Info: Calories: 143, Fat:4 g, Carbs:14 g, Protein:12 g, Sugars:0.8 g, Sodium:901 mg

Lemon Fat Bombs

Servings: 10

Cooking Time: 0 Minutes

Ingredients:

- Coconut butter, full-fat: 3/4 cup
- Avocado oil: 1/4 cup
- Lemon juice: 3 tablespoons
- Zest of lemon: 1
- Coconut cream, full-fat: 1 tablespoon
- Erythritol sweetener: 1 tablespoon
- Vanilla extract, unsweetened: 1 teaspoon
- Salt: 1/8 teaspoon

Directions:

1. Place all the ingredients for fat bombs in a blender and pulse until well combined.

2. Take a baking dish, line it with parchment sheet, then transfer the fat bomb mixture on the sheet and place the sheet into the freezer for 45 minutes until firm enough to shape into balls.

3. Then remove the baking sheet from the freezer, roll the fat bomb mixture into ten balls, and arrange the fat bombs on the baking sheet in a single layer.

4. Return the baking sheet into the freezer, let chilled until hard and set, and then store in the freezer for up to 2 months.

5. Serve when required.

Nutrition Info: Calories: 164 Fat: 16.7 g Protein: 1.3 g Net Carbs: 0.4 g Fiber: 3 g

Garden Patch Sandwiches On Multigrain Bread

Servings: 4

Cooking Time: 0 Minutes

Ingredients:

- 1pound extra-firm tofu, drained and patted dry
- 1 medium red bell pepper, finely chopped
- 1 celery rib, finely chopped
- 3 green onions, minced
- ¼ cup shelled sunflower seeds
- ½ cup vegan mayonnaise, homemade or store-bought
- ½ teaspoon salt
- ½ teaspoon celery salt
- ¼ teaspoon freshly ground black pepper

- 8 slices whole grain bread
- 4 (¼-inch) slices ripe tomato
- 4 lettuce leaves

Directions:

1. Preparing the Ingredients
2. Smash the tofu and place it in a large bowl. Add the bell pepper, celery, green onions, and sunflower seeds. Stir in the mayonnaise, salt, celery salt, and pepper and mix until well combined.
3. Finish and Serve
4. Toast the bread, if desired. Spread the mixture evenly onto 4 slices of the bread.

Nutrition Info: 166 Cal 15 g Fats 6.5 g Protein 2 g Net Carb 0 g Fiber

Sesame Almond Fat Bombs

Servings: 16

Cooking Time: 0 Minutes

Ingredients:

- 1 cup coconut oil
- 1 cup smooth almond butter
- ½ cup unsweetened cocoa powder
- ¼ cup almond flour
- Liquid stevia extract, to taste
- ½ cup toasted sesame seeds

Directions:

1. Combine the coconut oil and almond butter in a small saucepan.
2. Cook over low heat until melted, then whisk in the cocoa powder, almond flour, and liquid stevia.
3. Remove from heat and let cool until it hardens slightly.

4.   Divide the mixture into 16 even pieces
     and roll into balls.
5.   Roll the balls in the toasted sesame
     seeds and chill until ready to eat.

Nutrition Info: 260 calories 26g fat 4g protein
6g carbs 2g fiber 4g net carbs

Sugar Free Carrot Cake

Servings: 8

Cooking Time: 4 Hours

Ingredients:

- For Carrot cake:
- 2 eggs
- 1 1/2 almond flour
- 1/2 cup butter, melted
- ¼ cup heavy cream
- 1 teaspoon baking powder
- 1 teaspoon vanilla extract or almond extract, optional
- 1 cup sugar substitute
- 1 cup carrots, finely shredded
- 1 teaspoon cinnamon
- ¼ teaspoon nutmeg
- 1/8 teaspoon allspice
- 1 teaspoon ginger

- 1/2 teaspoon baking soda
- For cream cheese frosting:
- 1 cup confectioner's sugar substitute
- ¼ cup butter, softened
- 1 teaspoon almond extract
- 4 oz. cream cheese, softened

Directions:

1. Grease a loaf pan well and then set it aside.

2. Using a mixer, combine butter together with eggs, vanilla, sugar substitute and heavy cream in a mixing bowl, until well blended.

3. Combine almond flour together with baking powder, spices and the baking soda in a another bowl until well blended.

4. When done, combine the wet ingredients together with the dry ingredients until well blended, and then stir in carrots.

5. Pour the mixer into the prepared loaf
    pan, and then place the pan into a slow
    cooker on a trivet. Add 1 cup water
    inside.

6. Cook for about 4-5 hours on low. Be
    aware that the cake will be very moist.

7. When the cooking time is over, let the
    cake cool completely.

8. To prepare the cream cheese frosting:
    blend the cream cheese together with
    extract, butter and powdered sugar
    substitute until frosting is formed.

9. Top the cake with the frosting.

Nutrition Info: 299 calories; 25.4 g fat; 15 g
total carbs; 4 g protein

Spice Cake

Servings: 10

Cooking Time: 50 Minutes

Ingredients:

- Almond flour: 2 cups
- Erythritol sweetener: ½ cup
- Baking powder: 2 teaspoons
- Ground cinnamon: 1 teaspoon
- Ground ginger: 1 teaspoon
- Ground cloves: ¼ teaspoon
- Salt: ¼ teaspoon
- Eggs: 2
- Butter, unsalted, melted: 1/3 cup
- Water, divided: 1 1/3 cup
- Vanilla extract, unsweetened: ½ teaspoon
- Chopped toasted pecans: 3 tablespoons

Directions:

1. Place all the ingredients in a bowl, reserving 1 cup water and pecans, and stir well using a hand mixer until incorporated and a smooth batter comes together.

2. Take a 7-inch baking pan, spoon the batter on it, then smooth the top, sprinkle with pecans and cover the pan with aluminum foil.

3. Switch on the instant pot, pour in water, insert a trivet stand and place pan on it.

4. Shut the instant pot with its lid in the sealed position, then press the 'cake' button, press '+/-' to set the cooking time to 40 minutes and cook at high-pressure setting; when the pressure builds in the pot, the cooking timer will start.

5.   When the instant pot buzzes, press the 'keep warm' button, release pressure naturally for 10 minutes, then do a quick pressure release and open the lid.

6.   Take out the pan, uncover it, invert the pan on a plate to take out the cake and let cool for 10 minutes.

7.   Spread cream on top of the cake, then cut into slices and serve.

Nutrition Info: Calories: 229 Fat: 21 g Protein: 6 g Net Carbs: 2 g Fiber: 0 g

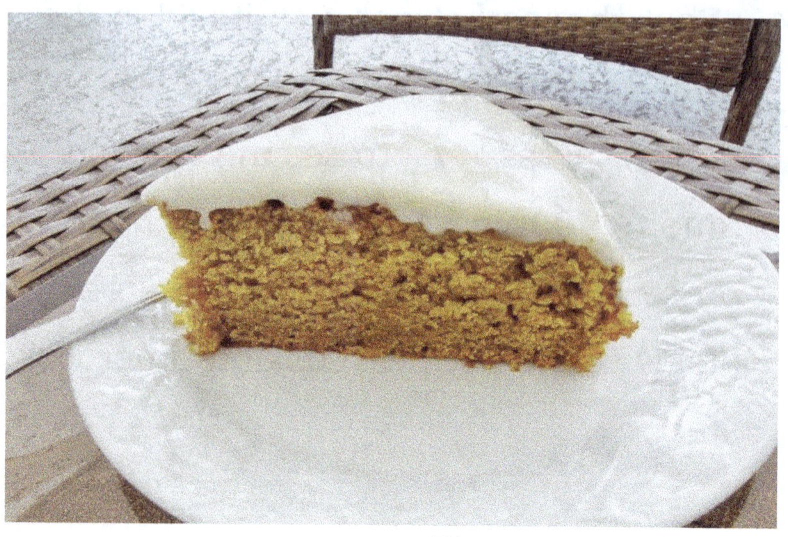

Creamy Chocolate Pie Ice Pops

Servings: 9

Cooking Time: 15 Minutes

Ingredients:

- 1 (4-serving size) package fat-free, sugar-free, reduced-calorie chocolate instant pudding mix
- 2 cups unsweetened almond milk or fat-free milk
- 1 cup frozen light whipped topping, thawed
- 1 oz. dark chocolate, melted
- 1 tbsp. crushed graham crackers

Directions:

1. Whisk together almond milk and pudding mix for 2 to 3 minutes in a medium bowl or until thick. Fold in whipped topping.

2. Ladle mixture into nine 3-oz. paper cups or ice pop molds. Insert sticks into the molds. In case you're using paper cups, use foil to cover each cup, make a small slit in the foil and then insert a wooden stick into each pop. Freeze overnight or until firm.

3. Unmold the pops. As you work with one pop at a time, drizzle with the melted chocolate and immediately sprinkle with graham crackers.

Nutrition Info: Calories: 60 calories; Total Carbohydrate: 9 g Cholesterol: 0 mg Total Fat: 3 g Fiber: 1 g Protein: 1 g Sodium: 175 mg Sugar: 2 g Saturated Fat: 2 g

Caramel Popcorn

Servings: 20

Cooking Time: 10 Minutes

Ingredients:

- 1 cup butter
- 2 cups brown sugar
- 1/2 cup corn syrup
- 1 tsp. salt
- 1/2 tsp. baking soda
- 1 tsp. vanilla extract
- 5 quarts popped popcorn

Directions:

1. Start preheating the oven to 250°F (95°C). In a very big bowl, put popcorn.

2. Melt butter over medium heat in a medium-sized saucepan. Mix in salt, corn syrup, and brown sugar. Boil it,

tossing continually. Boil without tossing for 4 minutes. Take away from the heat and mix in vanilla and soda. Add to the popcorn in a thin flow, tossing to blend.

3. Put in 2 big shallow cookie sheets and bake in the preheated oven for 1 hour, tossing every 15 minutes. Take out of the oven and let cool fully and then crumble into chunks.

Nutrition Info: Calories: 253 calories Total Carbohydrate: 32.8 g Cholesterol: 24 mg Total Fat: 14 g Protein: 0.9 g Sodium: 340 mg

Tiramisu Shots

Servings: 4

Cooking Time: 10 Minutes

Ingredients:

- 1 pack silken tofu
- 1 oz. dark chocolate, finely chopped
- ¼ cup sugar substitute
- 1 teaspoon lemon juice
- ¼ cup brewed espresso
- Pinch salt
- 24 slices angel food cake
- Cocoa powder (unsweetened)

Directions:

1. Add tofu, chocolate, sugar substitute, lemon juice, espresso and salt in a food processor.
2. Pulse until smooth.

3. Add angel food cake pieces into shot glasses.

4. Drizzle with the cocoa powder.

5. Pour the tofu mixture on top.

6. Top with the remaining angel food cake pieces.

7. Chill for 30 minutes and serve.

Nutrition Info: Calories 75 Total Fat 1.8 g Total Carbohydrate 12 g Protein 2.9 g

Fruit Kebab

Servings: 12

Cooking Time: 0 Minutes

Ingredients:

- 3 apples
- ¼ cup orange juice
- 1 ½ lb. watermelon
- ¾ cup blueberries

Directions:

1. Use a star-shaped cookie cutter to cut out stars from the apple and watermelon.
2. Soak the apple stars in orange juice.
3. Thread the apple stars, watermelon stars and blueberries into skewers.
4. Refrigerate for 30 minutes before serving.

Nutrition Info: Calories 52 Total Fat 0 g Saturated Fat 0 g Cholesterol 0 mg Sodium 1 mg Total Carbohydrate 14 g Dietary Fiber 2 g Total Sugars 10 g Protein 1 g Potassium 134 mg

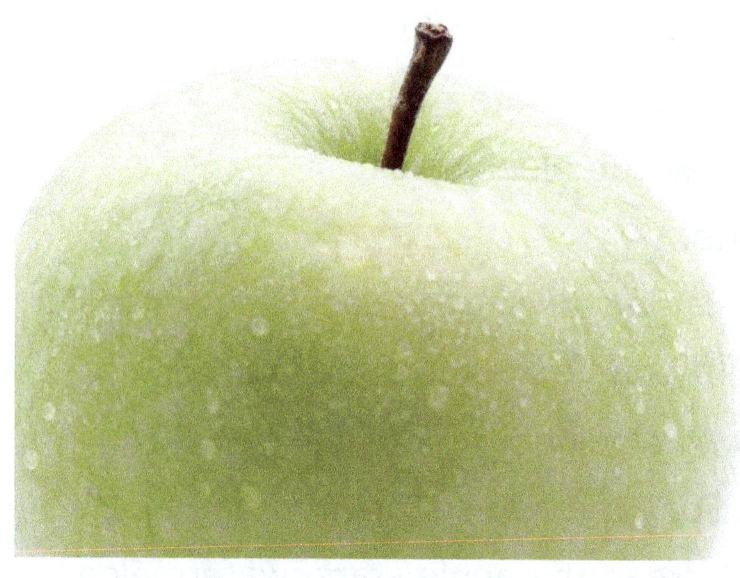

Cheese Berry Fat Bomb

Servings: 12

Cooking Time: 5 Minutes

Ingredients:

- 1 cup fresh berries, wash
- 1/2 cup coconut oil
- 1 1/2 cup cream cheese, softened
- 1 tbsp vanilla
- 2 tbsp swerve

Directions:

1. Add all ingredients to the blender and blend until smooth and combined.
2. Spoon mixture into small candy molds and refrigerate until set.
3. Serve and enjoy.

Nutrition Info: Calories 175 Fat 17 g Carbohydrates 2 g Sugar 1 g Protein 2.1 g Cholesterol 29 mg

Tamari Toasted Almonds

Servings: ½

Cooking Time: 8 Minutes

Ingredients:

- ½ cup raw almonds, or sunflower seeds
- 2 tablespoons tamari, or soy sauce
- 1 teaspoon toasted sesame oil

Directions:

1. Preparing the Ingredients
2. Heat a dry skillet to medium-high heat, then add the almonds, stirring frequently to keep them from burning. Once the almonds are toasted—7-8 minutes for almonds, or 34 minutes for sunflower seeds—pour the tamari and

sesame oil into the hot skillet and stir to coat.

3. You can turn off the heat, and as the almonds cool the tamari mixture will stick and dry on to the nuts.

Nutrition Info: Calories: 89 Total fat: 8g Carbs: 3g Fiber: 2g Protein: 4g

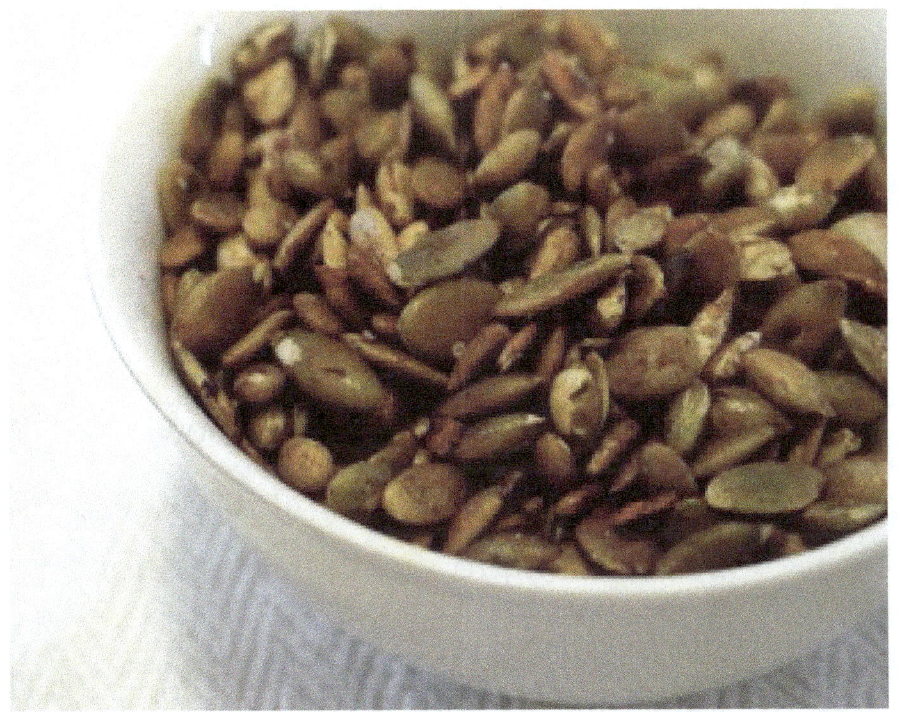

Choco Peppermint Cake

Servings: 4

Cooking Time: 10 Minutes

Ingredients:

- Cooking spray
- ⅓ cup oil
- 15 oz. package chocolate cake mix
- 3 eggs, beaten
- 1 cup water
- ¼ teaspoon peppermint extract

Directions:

1. Spray slow cooker with oil.
2. Mix all the ingredients in a bowl.
3. Use an electric mixer on medium speed setting to mix ingredients for 2 minutes.
4. Pour mixture into the slow cooker.

5. Cover the pot and cook on low for 3 hours.

6. Let cool before slicing and serving.

Nutrition Info: Calories 185 Total Fat 7.4 g Total Carbohydrate 27 g Protein 3.8 g

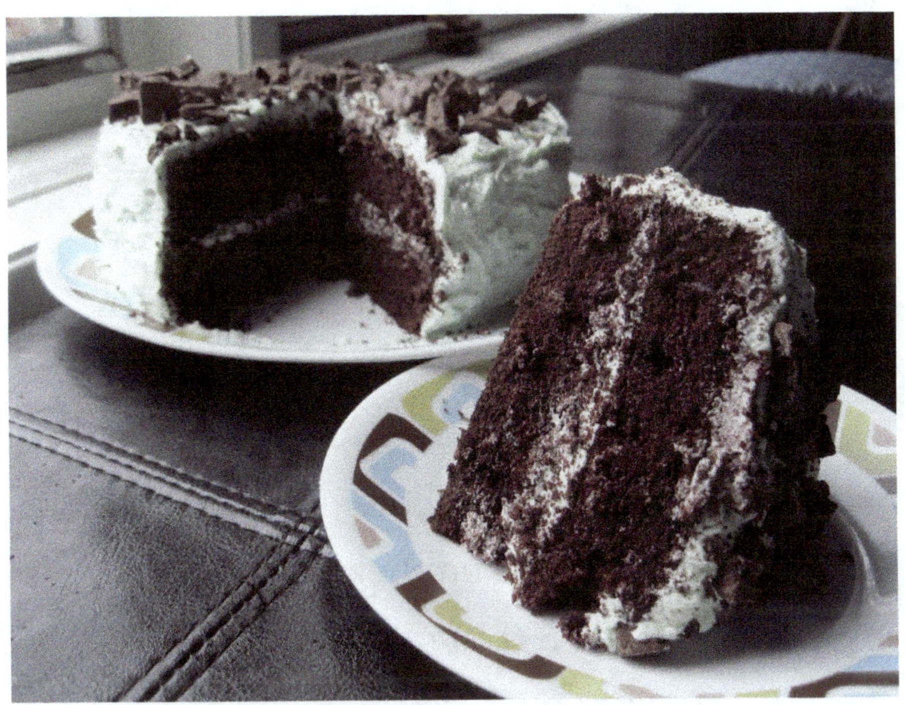

Frozen Lemon & Blueberry

Servings: 4

Cooking Time: 10 Minutes

Ingredients:

- 6 cup fresh blueberries
- 8 sprigs fresh thyme
- ¾ cup light brown sugar
- 1 teaspoon lemon zest
- ¼ cup lemon juice
- 2 cups water

Directions:

1. Add blueberries, thyme and sugar in a pan over medium heat.
2. Cook for 6 to 8 minutes.
3. Transfer mixture to a blender.
4. Remove thyme sprigs.
5. Stir in the remaining ingredients.
6. Pulse until smooth.

7. Strain mixture and freeze for 1 hour.

Nutrition Info: Calories 78 Total Fat 0 g Total Carbohydrate 20 g Protein 3 g

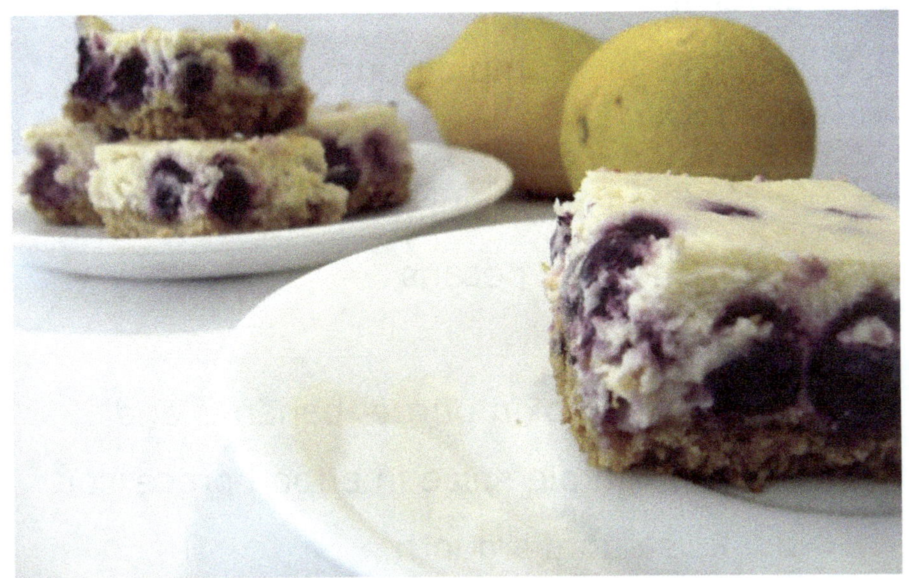

Pumpkin & Banana Ice Cream

Servings: 4

Cooking Time: 10 Minutes

Ingredients:

- 15 oz. pumpkin puree
- 4 bananas, sliced and frozen
- 1 teaspoon pumpkin pie spice
- Chopped pecans

Directions:

1. Add pumpkin puree, bananas and pumpkin pie spice in a food processor.
2. Pulse until smooth.
3. Chill in the refrigerator.
4. Garnish with pecans.

Nutrition Info: Calories 71 Total Fat 0.4 g Total Carbohydrate 18 g Protein 1.2 g

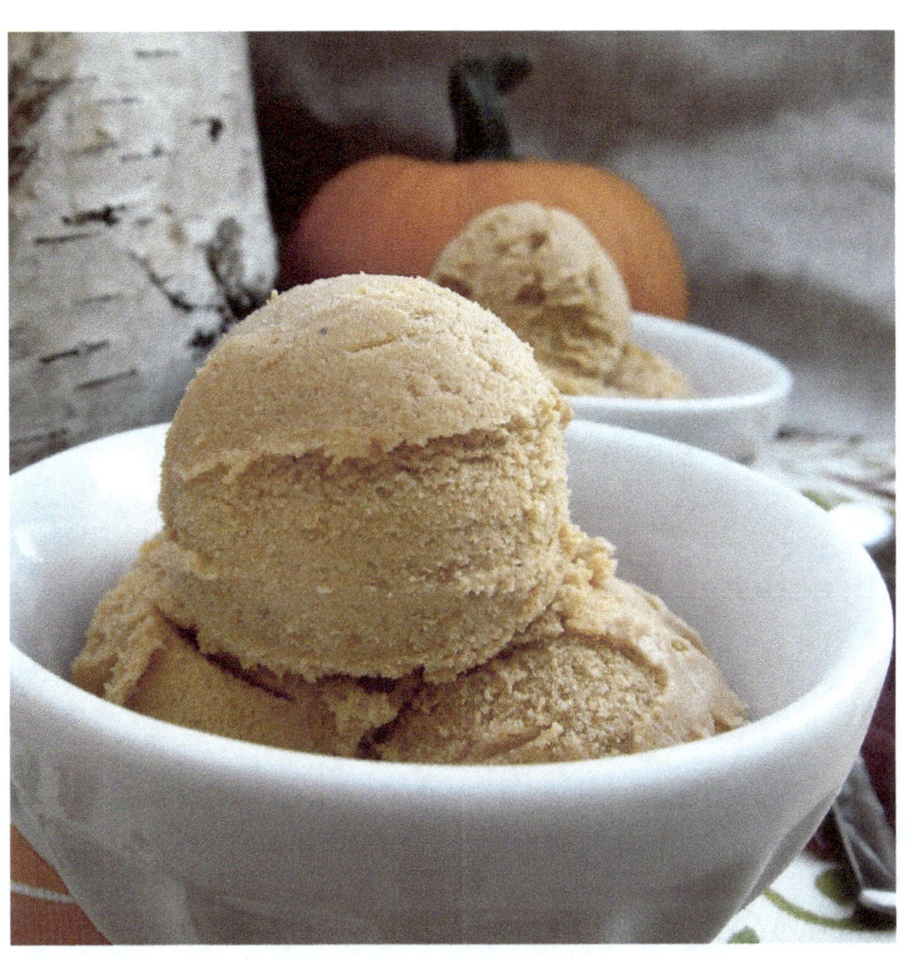

Coconut Chia Pudding

Servings: 6

Cooking Time: 0 Minutes

Ingredients:

- 2 ¼ cup canned coconut milk
- 1 teaspoon vanilla extract
- Pinch salt
- ½ cup chia seeds

Directions:

1. Combine the coconut milk, vanilla, and salt in a bowl.
2. Stir well and sweeten with stevia to taste.
3. Whisk in the chia seeds and chill overnight.
4. Spoon into bowls and serve with chopped nuts or fruit.

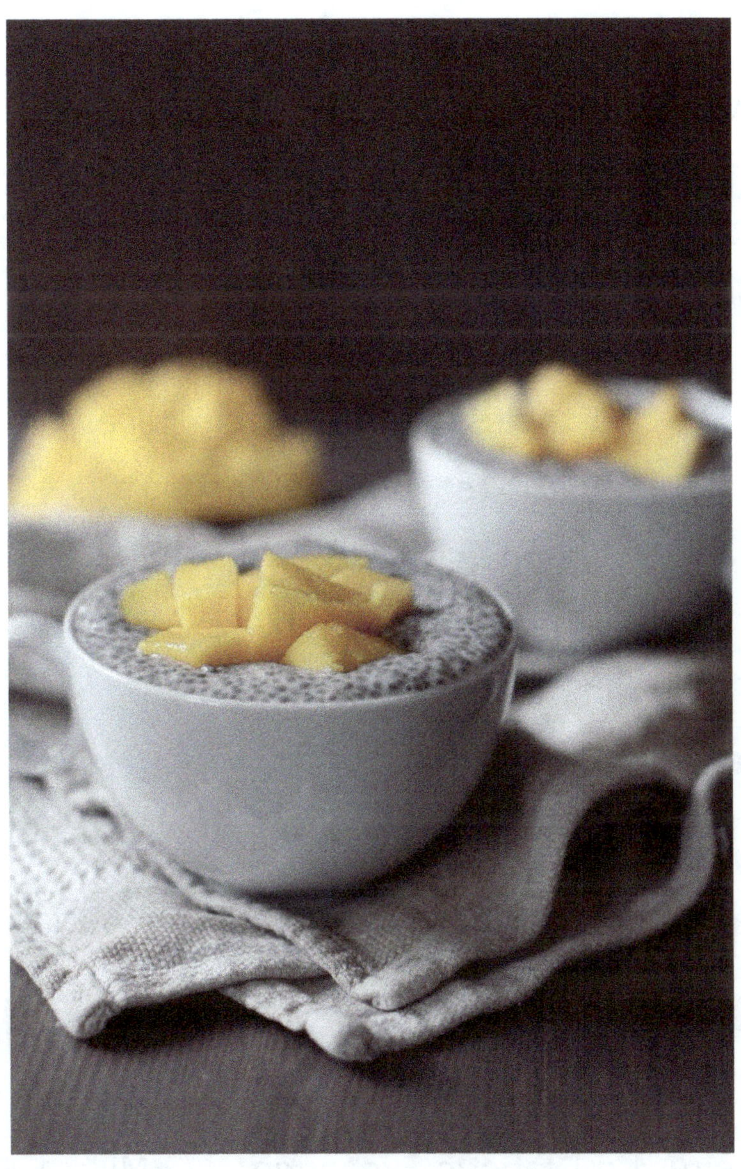

Strawberries In Honey Yogurt Dip

Servings: 4

Cooking Time: 0 Minutes

Ingredients:

- 1 cup plain yogurt, low-fat
- 1 tablespoon of orange juice
- 1 to 2 teaspoons of honey
- Ground cinnamon
- 1 quart of fresh strawberries (remove stems)

Directions:

1. Combine first four ingredients to make a sauce. Pour over strawberries and serve.

Nutrition Info: Calories: 88 Carbohydrates: 16 g Fiber: 4 g Fats: 1 g Sodium: 41 mg Protein: 4 g Diabetic Exchange: 1/2 Milk, 1 Fruit

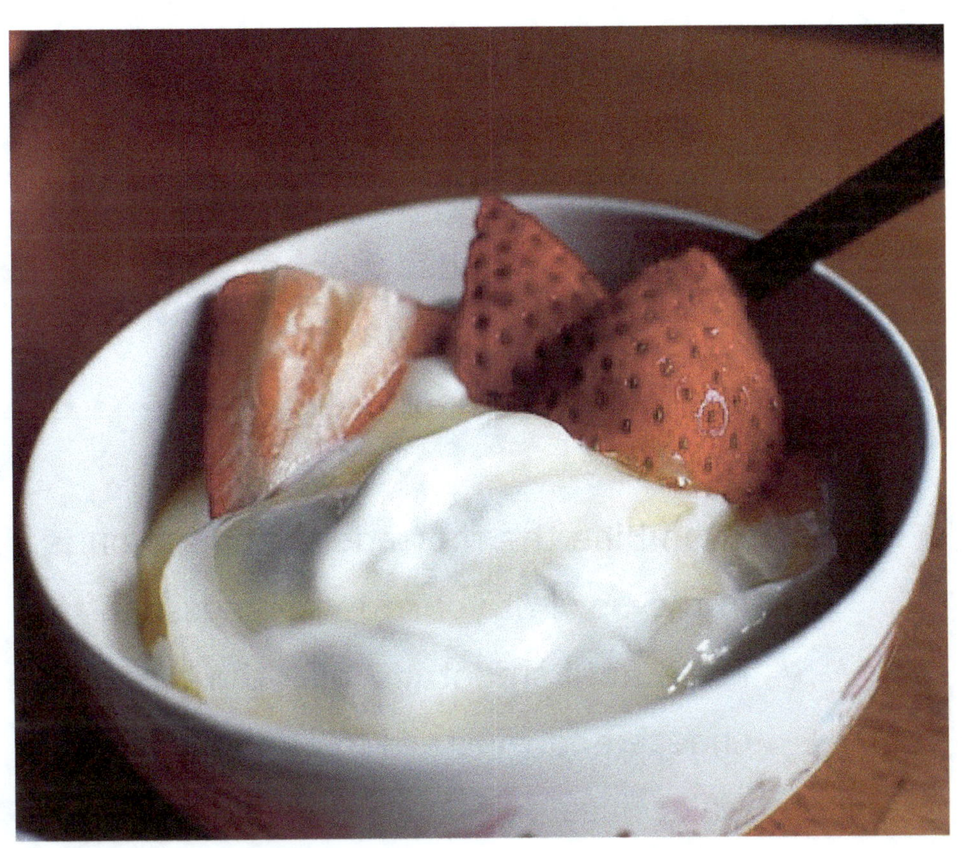

Mortadella & Bacon Balls

Servings: 2

Cooking Time: 20 Minutes

Ingredients:

- 4 ounces Mortadella sausage
- 4 bacon slices, cooked and crumbled
- 2 tbsp almonds, chopped
- ½ tsp Dijon mustard
- 3 ounces' cream cheese

Directions:

1. Combine the mortadella and almonds in the bowl of your food processor. Pulse until smooth. Whisk the cream cheese and mustard in another bowl. Make balls out of the mortadella mixture.

2. Make a thin cream cheese layer over. Coat with bacon, arrange on a plate and chill before serving.

Nutrition Info: Calories 547 Fat: 51g Net Carbs: 3.4g Protein: 21.5g

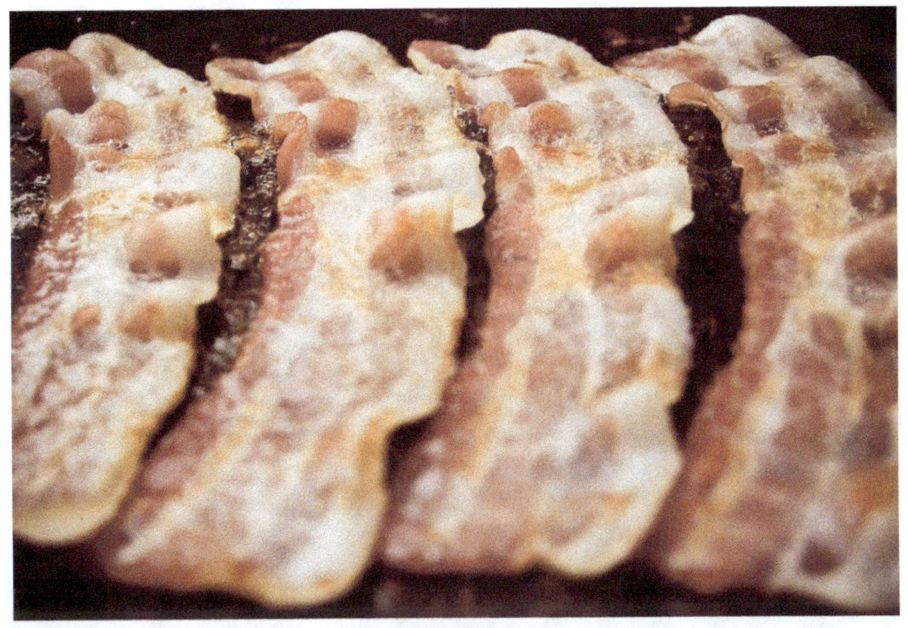

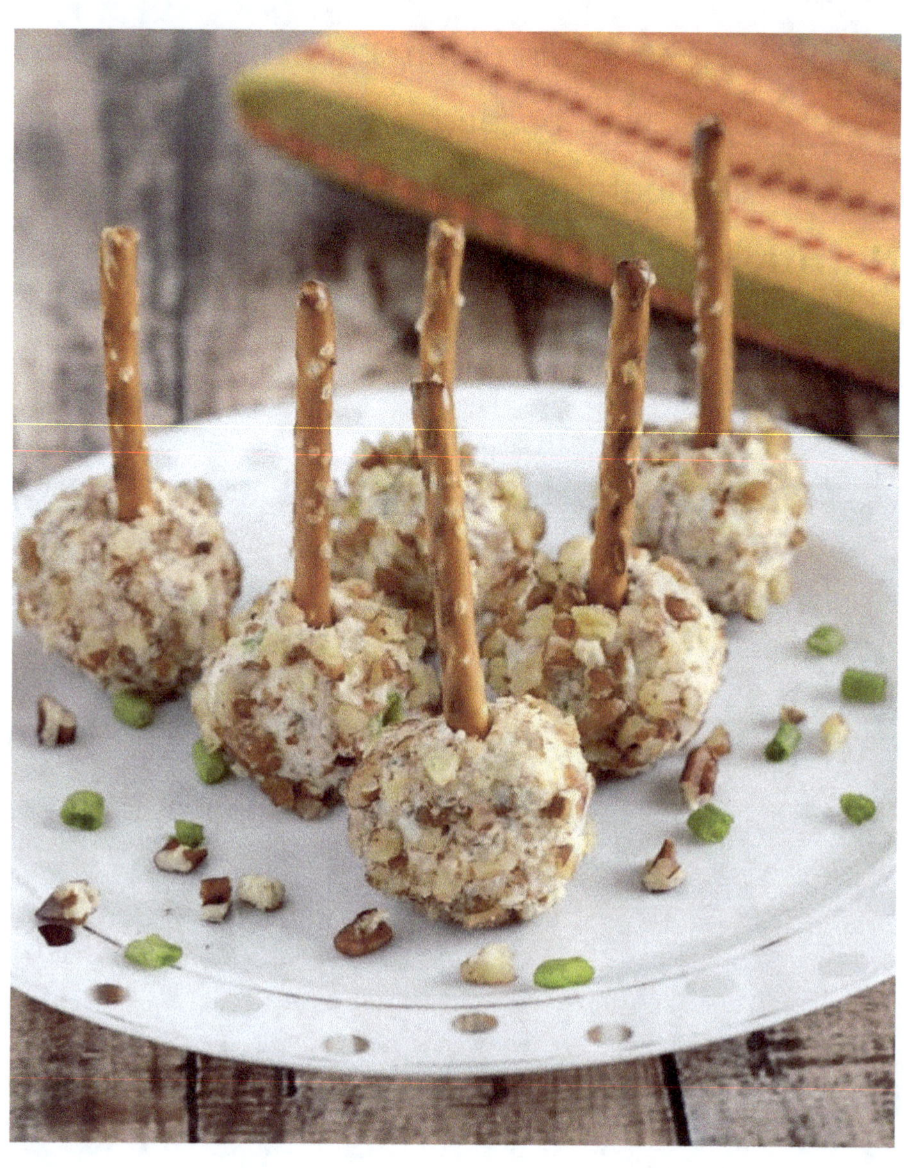

Lemon Cake

Servings: 9

Cooking Time: 20 Minutes

Ingredients:

- 2 Medium lemons
- 4 Large eggs
- 2 Tablespoons of almond butter
- 2 Tablespoons of avocado oil
- 1/3 cup of coconut flour
- 4-5 tablespoons of honey (or another sweetener of your choice)
- 1/2 tablespoon of baking soda

Directions:

1. Preheat your oven to a temperature of about 350 F.
2. Crack the eggs in a large bowl and set two egg whites aside.

3. Whisk the 2 whites of eggs with the egg yolks, the honey, the oil, the almond butter, the lemon zest and the juice and whisk very well together.

4. Combine the baking soda with the coconut flour and gradually add this dry mixture to the wet ingredients and keep whisking for a couple of minutes.

5. Beat the two eggs with a hand mixer and beat the egg into foam.

6. Add the white egg foam gradually to the mixture with a silicone spatula.

7. Transfer your obtained batter to tray covered with a baking paper.

8. Bake your cake for about 20 to 22 minutes.

9. Let the cake cool for 5 minutes; then slice your cake.

10. Serve and enjoy your delicious cake!

Nutrition Info: Calories: 164| Fat: 12g | Carbohydrates: 7.1 | Fiber: 2.7g |Protein: 10.9g

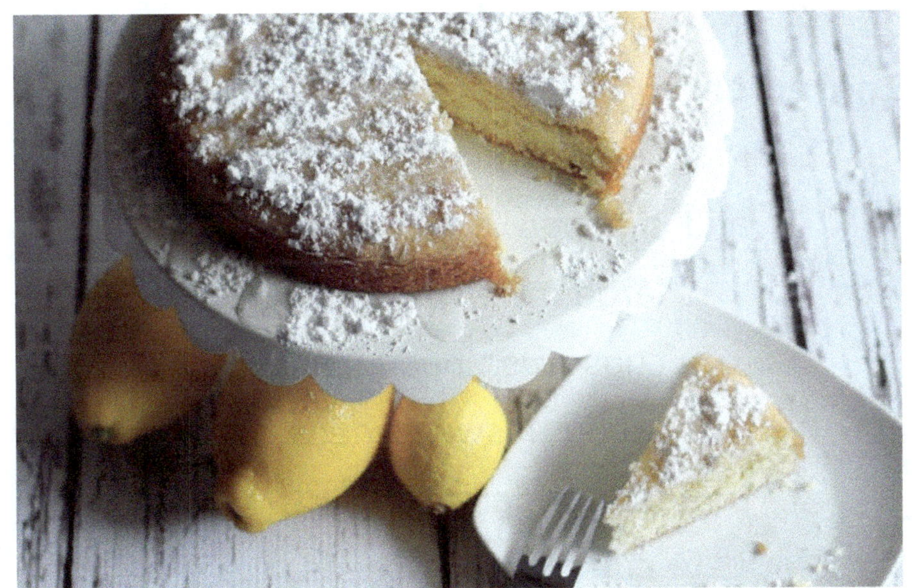

Green Fruity Smoothie

Servings: 2

Cooking Time: 10 Minutes

Ingredients:

- 1 cup frozen mango, peeled, pitted, and chopped
- 1 large frozen banana, peeled
- 2 cups fresh baby spinach
- 1 scoop unsweetened vegan vanilla protein powder
- ¼ cup pumpkin seeds
- 2 tablespoons hemp hearts
- 1½ cups unsweetened almond milk

Directions:

1. In a high-speed blender, place all the ingredients and pulse until creamy.
2. Pour into two glasses and serve immediately.

Nutrition Info: Calories 355 Total Fat 16.1 g
Saturated Fat 2.4 g Cholesterol 0 mg Sodium
295 mg Total Carbs 34.6 g Fiber 6.2 g Sugar
19.9 g Protein 23.4 g

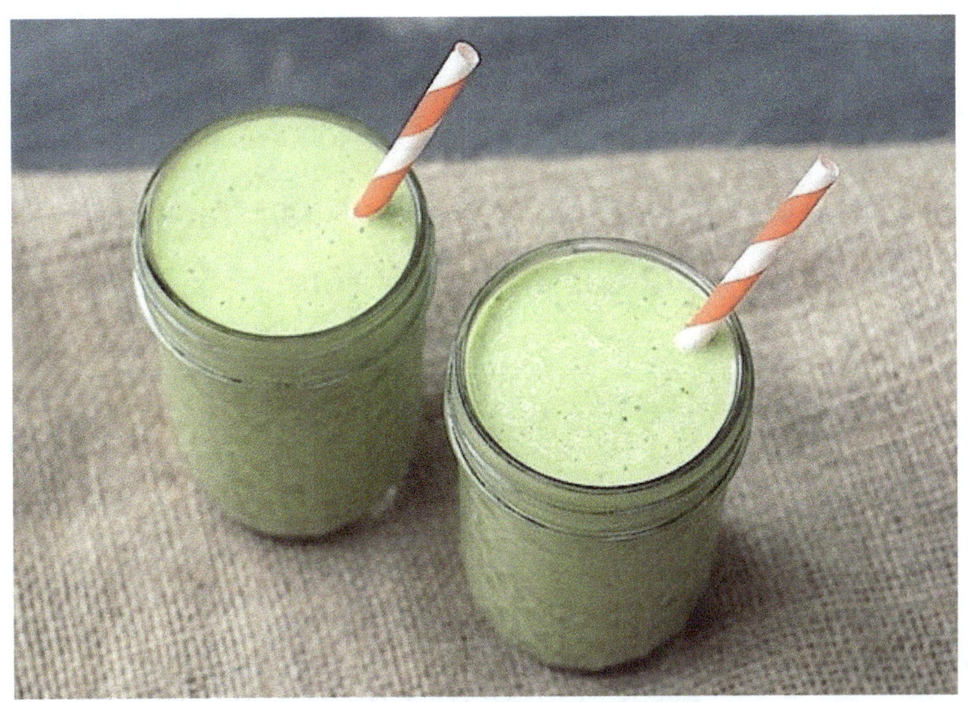

Baked Creamy Custard With Maple

Servings: 6

Cooking Time: 15 Minutes

Ingredients:

- 2 1/2 cups half-and-half, fat-free
- 1/2 cup egg substitute, cholesterol-free
- 1/4 cup sugar
- 2 teaspoons vanilla
- Dash ground nutmeg
- 3 cups of boiling water
- 2 tablespoons of maple syrup

Directions:

1. Spray 6 ramekins or custard cups with light non-stick cooking spray. Preheat your oven to 325ºF.

2. Combine first five ingredients and mix well. Pour into your ramekins.

3. Pour the boiling water in a 13x9-inch baking dish. Place the ramekins in the dish and bake 1 hour 15 minutes.

4. Cool the ramekins on a cooling rack. Cover with a plastic wrap and chill in the fridge overnight.

5. Drizzle with maple syrup before serving.

Nutrition Info: Calories: 131 Carbohydrates: 23 g Fiber: 0 g Fats: 1 g Sodium: 139 mg Protein: 5 g

Lemon Cookies

Servings: 6

Cooking Time: 12 Minutes

Ingredients:

- ¼ cup unsweetened applesauce
- 1 cup cashew butter
- 1 teaspoon fresh lemon zest, grated finely
- 2 tablespoons fresh lemon juice
- Pinch of sea salt

Directions:

1. Preheat the oven to 350 degrees F. Line a large cookie sheet with parchment paper.
2. In a food processor, add all ingredients and pulse until smooth.

3. With a tablespoon, place the mixture onto prepared cookie sheet in a single layer.

4. Bake for about 12 minutes or until golden brown.

5. Remove from oven and place the cookie sheet onto a wire rack to cool for about 5 minutes.

6. Carefully invert the cookies onto wire rack to cool completely before serving.

7. Meal Prep Tip: Store these cookies in an airtight container, by placing parchment papers between the cookies to avoid the sticking. These cookies can be stored in the refrigerator for up to 2 weeks.

Nutrition Info: Calories 257 Total Fat 21.9 g Saturated Fat 4.2 g Cholesterol 0 mg Total Carbs 13.1 g Sugar 1.2 g Fiber 1 g Sodium 47 mg Potassium 248 mg Protein 7.6 g

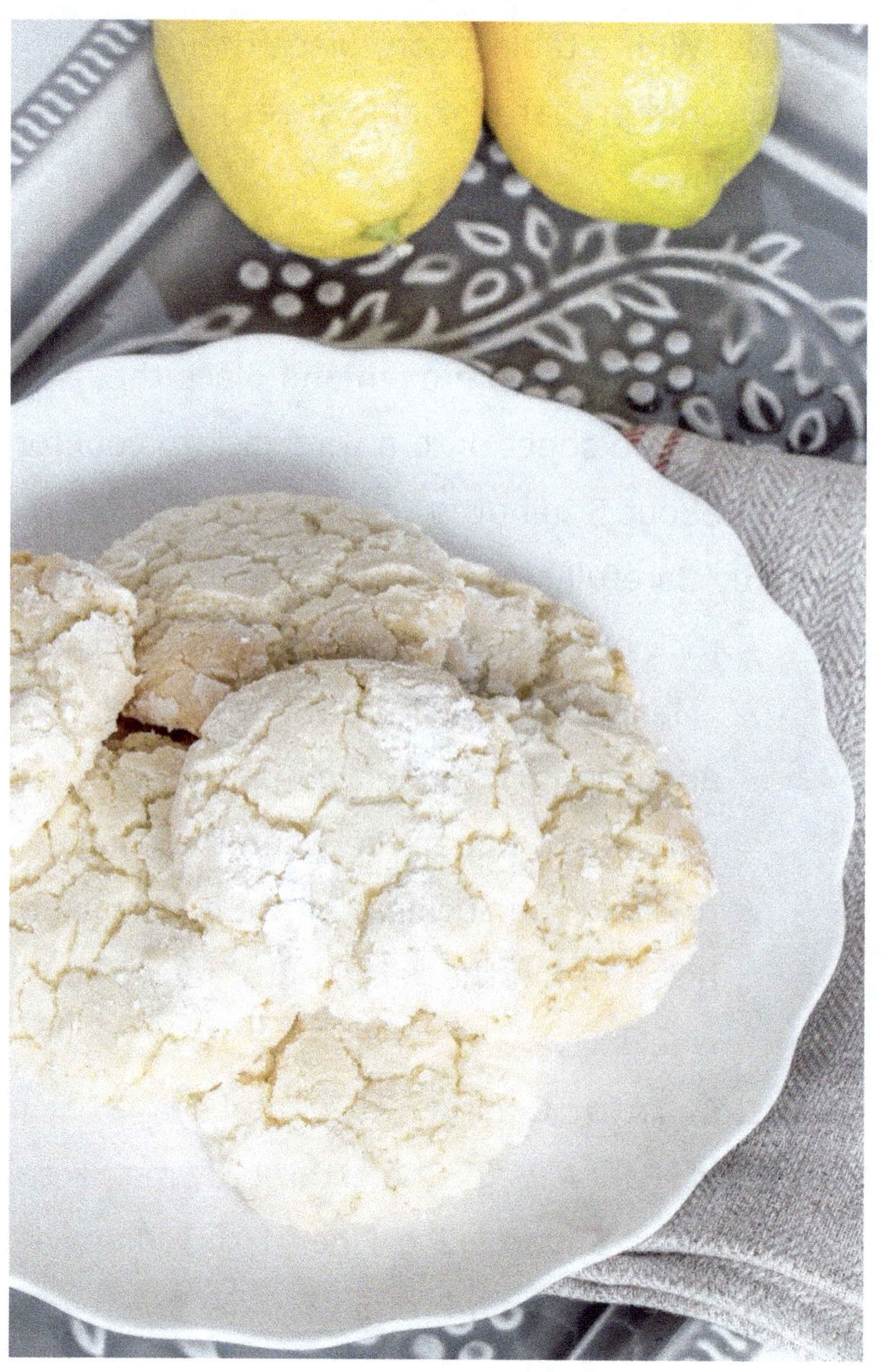

Pineapple Nice Cream

Servings: 6

Cooking Time: 15 Minutes

Ingredients:

- 1 16-oz. package frozen pineapple chunks
- 1 cup frozen mango chunks or 1 large mango, peeled, seeded and chopped
- 1 tbsp. lemon juice or lime juice

Directions:

1. In a food processor, process the mango, lemon or lime juice, and pineapple until creamy and smooth. You can add a 1/4 cup of water if the mango is frozen. Serve it immediately if you want to have the best texture.

Nutrition Info: Calories: 55 calories; Total Carbohydrate: 14 g Cholesterol: 0 mg Total

Fat: 0 g Fiber: 2 g Protein: 1 g Sodium: 1 mg
Sugar: 11 g Saturated Fat: 0 g

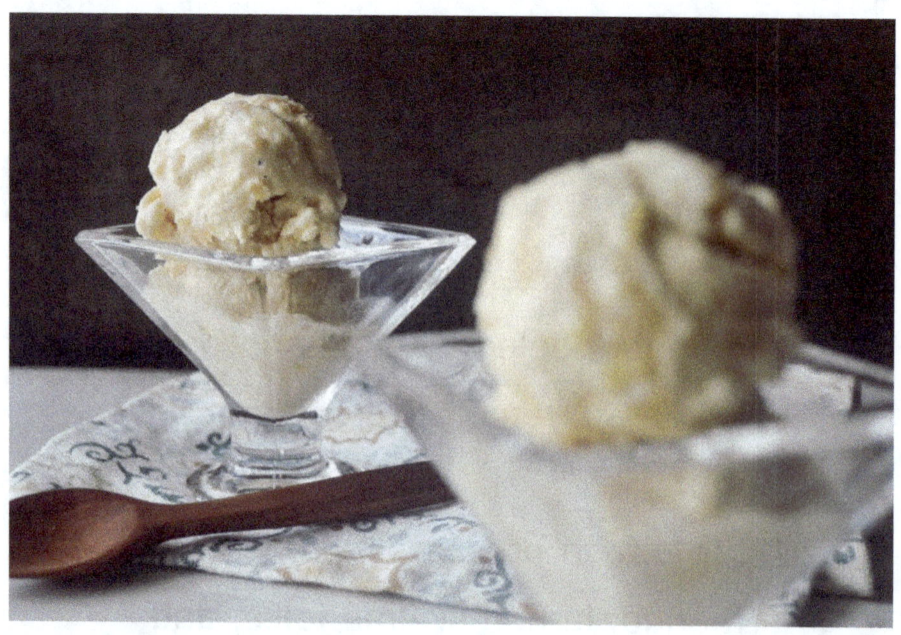

9 781801 908979